GREEN SMOOTHIE REVOLUTION

Transform Your Body in Just 10 Days!

Written By David Hanson

Table of Contents

Introduction

lcome to "Green Smoothie Revolution: Transform Your dy in Just 10 Days!" This book is your guide to bracing the incredible benefits of green smoothies and ieving a healthier, more vibrant lifestyle.

roduction: Embrace the Power of Green Smoothies In s introduction, we invite you to embark on a life-anging journey fueled by the power of green smoothies. cover how these nutrient-packed beverages can nsform your body and enhance your overall well-being.

apter 1: The World of Green Smoothies In Chapter 1, delve into the world of green smoothies, exploring what ey are and the multitude of health benefits they offer. om improved digestion to weight loss support and reased energy levels, you'll uncover the reasons why en smoothies are a fantastic addition to any lifestyle.

Chapter 2: Getting Started with Green Smoothies Chap
2 is your gateway to the world of green smoothies. G
essential knowledge on selecting the right ingredients
delicious and nourishing blends. We'll also prov
guidance on the necessary tools, preparation techniqu
and storage methods to ensure your green smoothies
both fresh and convenient.

Chapter 3: The 10-Day Transformation Chapter 3 is t
heart of our journey, where we embark on a 10-c
transformational experience. Each day, you'll disco
carefully curated green smoothie recipes accompanied
insights into their unique benefits. From energiz
morning blends to soothing evening elixirs, these recip
will guide you toward a renewed sense of vitality.

Chapter 4: Beyond the 10-Day Challenge in Chapter 4,
go beyond the initial 10-day challenge and explore how
incorporate green smoothies into your regular lifesty

cover new flavors, variations, and ways to customize
ur smoothies to suit your dietary needs. Whether you're
gan, gluten-free, or have specific nutritional
uirements, this chapter has you covered.

nclusion: Embrace the Green Smoothie Revolution. In
nclusion, "Green Smoothie Revolution: Transform Your
dy in Just 10 Days!" is your ticket to a healthier and
re vibrant life.

t ready to embark on a delicious and transformative
rney that will leave you feeling revitalized, energized,
d ready to conquer the world. Embrace the
raordinary power of green smoothies and unlock the
ential within you.

e you ready to revolutionize your health and well-being?
's dive into the world of green smoothies and embark
this incredible journey together!

Chapter 1: The Power of Green Smoothies

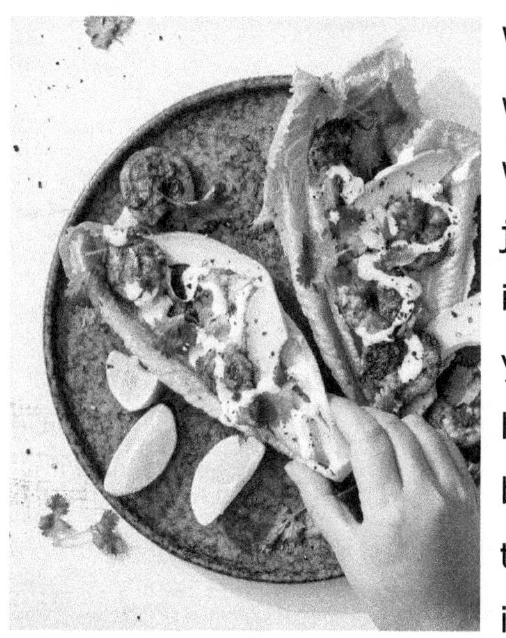

Welcome to the captivat[ing] world of green smoothi[es] where we will embark o[n a] journey to discover th[e] incredible power to transf[orm] your body and enhance y[our] health. Prepare to be ama[zed] by the boundless possibilit[ies] that lie ahead as we de[lve] into the realm of gr[een] smoothies.

1.0 Unveiling the Magic of Green Smoothies

In this chapter, we will unravel the secrets behind [the] enchanting green smoothies. We will explore their uni[que] composition, dissecting the key ingredients that m[ake] them extraordinary. From nutrient-rich leafy greens

cious fruits and other essential components, you will
n a deep understanding of what makes green smoothies
ly special.

1 Decoding the Green Smoothie Formula

:'s begin by unraveling the mysteries of the green
oothie formula. We will delve into the precise
mbination of ingredients that make up these vibrant
ncoctions. Discover the art of selecting the perfect leafy
eens, fruits, and other nourishing elements to create
icious and healthful blends.

2 The Abundance of Benefits

this section, we will explore the multitude of benefits
at green smoothies offer. Prepare to be astonished as
discuss the myriad ways in which these vibrant elixirs
n positively impact your overall well-being. From
creased energy levels and improved digestion to weight
anagement support and a strengthened immune system,

green smoothies provide an abundance of hea
advantages.

1.3 Transforming Your Body from Within

In the following pages, we will dive even deeper into t
transformative effects of green smoothies on your bod
Uncover the remarkable nutrients and compounds fou
within green smoothie ingredients that promote optim
health. Learn how these elements work synergistically
boost vitality, nourish your skin, enhance mental clari
and support detoxification processes.

Furthermore, we will explore the long-term impact
incorporating green smoothies into your daily routir
Discover how these vibrant beverages can help you bre
unhealthy habits, increase your intake of fruits a
vegetables, and cultivate a mindful approach to mealtim

oughout this chapter, we aim to provide you with the

ential knowledge and inspiration to understand why

en smoothies have the potential to revolutionize your

l-being. Get ready to embrace the transformative

wer of green smoothies and embark on a personal

rney of self-improvement.

member, with each sip of a green smoothie, you are

rishing your body and taking a step toward a healthier

d more vibrant version of yourself. So, let's embark on

s adventure together, unraveling the full potential of

en smoothies and experiencing the remarkable benefits

y bring.

Chapter 2: Getting Started with Green Smoothies

In this chapter, we will lay the foundation for your gre
smoothie journey by providing you with practical guidar
on how to get started with creating and enjoying delicic
green smoothies. From choosing the right ingredients
essential equipment and preparation techniques, yo
have all the tools you need to kick-start your gre
smoothie adventure.

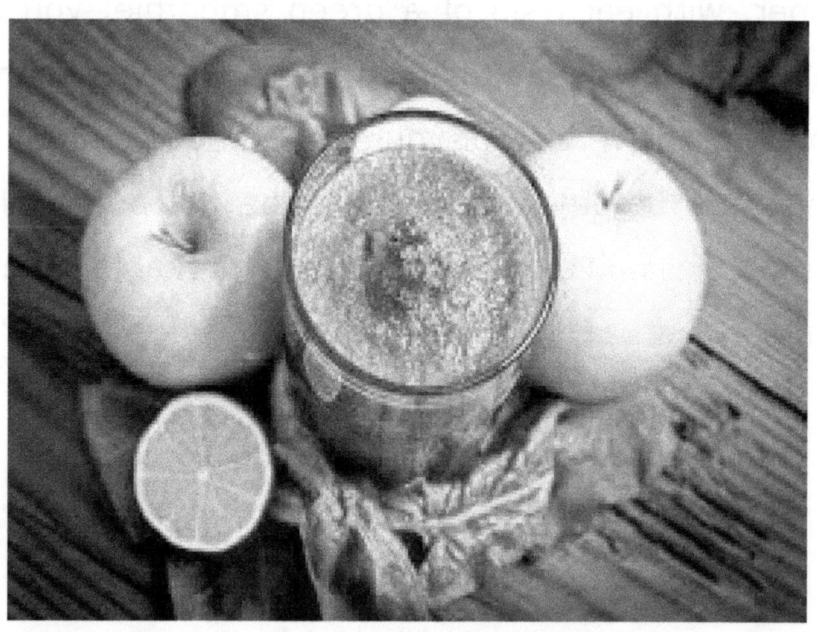

Choosing the Right Ingredients

The key to a successful green smoothie lies in selecting the right ingredients. In this section, we will guide you through the process of choosing the freshest and most nutrient-dense fruits and leafy greens for your smoothies. We'll explore the benefits of different types of greens, such as spinach, kale, and Swiss chard, and discuss how to incorporate a variety of fruits to add flavor and natural sweetness. You'll also discover the importance of organic produce and tips for sourcing high-quality ingredients.

Essential Equipment for Green Smoothie Making

To create smooth and creamy green smoothies, you'll need the right equipment. In this section, we'll discuss the essential tools you'll need, such as blenders and juicers, and provide insights into choosing the best options for your budget and needs. We'll also cover additional accessories that can enhance your green smoothie experience, such as reusable straws and storage containers.

2.3 Preparing and Storing Green Smoothies

Efficiency is key when it comes to incorporating gre
smoothies into your daily routine. In this section, w
share practical tips and techniques for preparing y
smoothies quickly and easily. You'll learn about prepp
ingredients in advance, creating smoothie packs
convenience, and using proper blending techniques
achieve the desired consistency.

We'll also discuss proper storage methods to ensure
freshness and flavor of your green smoothies, whether y
plan to enjoy them immediately or save some for later.

By the end of this chapter, you'll have a solid foundat
in selecting the right ingredients, acquiring the necess
equipment, and efficiently preparing and storing y
green smoothies. You'll be ready to embark on your
day green smoothie transformation journey w

fidence. So, let's get started and unlock the potential
these vibrant and nutritious beverages!

member, creating a green smoothie is not only about
urishing your body but also about having fun and
ploring new flavors. Get ready to blend your way to a
althier you!

GREEN SMOOTHIE REVOLUTION

Chapter 3: The 10-Day Green Smoothie Transformation

Welcome to the exciting 10-day green smoot[h]
transformation journey! In this chapter, we will focus [on]
revitalizing your body and introducing you to the incredi[ble]
benefits of incorporating a daily green smoothie into yo[ur]
life. Prepare to be amazed as you discover a new reci[pe]
each day, carefully crafted to enhance your overall hea[lth]
and well-being. Get ready to experience a life-alteri[ng]
transformation through the power of green smoothies.

3.1 Preparing for the 10-Day Challenge

Success begins with proper preparation. In this section, [we]
will provide you with valuable insights on how to g[et]
emotionally and physically ready for the upcoming 10-d[ay]
challenge. Learn how to create a schedule that allows [for]
regular green smoothie consumption, set realistic goa[ls]
and create a supportive environment. We will also addre[ss]
common challenges and offer practical advice to help y[ou]
overcome any obstacles along the way.

2 Daily Green Smoothie Recipes

e heart of the 10-day challenge lies in the daily green oothie recipes. These recipes are carefully designed to urish your body and unlock specific benefits. In the owing paragraphs, you will find a diverse selection of uthwatering and nutritious blends that will leave you ling revitalized, energized, and satisfied. Each recipe hlights key ingredients and their unique health vantages. Whether you need a morning boost or support a peaceful night's sleep, there's a wide variety of vors and benefits to explore.

t ready to embark on an incredible 10-day journey of nsformation with green smoothies as your guide. Each brings you closer to a healthier and more vibrant rsion of yourself.

Let's embrace the potential of green smoothies a
embark on this remarkable adventure together.

Let me provide you with a glimpse of what awaits you:

Day 1: Revitalizing Morning Starter Smoothi

Kickstart your day with a nutrient-packed smoothie t
will energize and invigorate you, setting the tone fo
productive morning.

Day 2: Green Cleanse and Detox Smoothie

Experience a refreshing and detoxifying green smoot
that will leave you feeling rejuvenated and revitalized.

Day 3: Immunity-Boosting Power Drink

Boost your immune system with a delicious blend
immune-boosting ingredients that will support your over
health and well-being.

y 4: Digestive Health Soother Smoothie

ure your digestive system with a soothing and
rishing smoothie that promotes a healthy gut and
roved digestion.

y 5: Weight Loss Green Elixir

elerate your weight loss journey with a nutrient-dense
en elixir specially formulated to support your weight
s goals.

y 6: Radiant Skin Glow Smoothie

ieve a radiant and glowing complexion by nourishing
r skin from within with a smoothie packed with
ioxidants and nutrients.

Day 7: Muscle Recovery Refuel Smoothie

Replenish your muscles and aid in their recovery with protein-rich smoothie that will help you bounce back af workouts.

Day 8: Mental Clarity and Focus Smoothie

Enhance your cognitive abilities and sharpen your men clarity and focus with a smoothie packed with bra boosting nutrients.

Day 9: Heart-Healthy Bliss Smoothie

Take care of your heart health with a delightful smoot that supports cardiovascular function and promotes healthy heart.

ay 10: Relaxation and Sleep-Inducing noothie

wind and prepare for a restful night's sleep with a ming smoothie that promotes relaxation and tranquility.

t ready to embark on an exhilarating journey of nsformation, where each day brings a delightful and tritious smoothie to enhance your overall health. Allow ese green smoothies to nurture your well-being and pire a happier and healthier version of yourself.

the end of this chapter, you'll have completed a 10-day een smoothie transformation, feeling revitalized and uipped with a newfound appreciation for the power of een smoothies. The journey doesn't end here, though! apter 4 will guide you on how to incorporate green oothies into your long-term lifestyle and explore further riations and adaptations.

Get ready to embark on a transformative journey that will leave you amazed by the remarkable changes that can occur in just 10 days. Cheers to your health and well being!

Remember, each day brings you closer to a healthier and more vibrant you. So, let's raise our green smoothie glasses and toast to a radiant transformation!

To kickstart your 10-day green smoothie transformation, begin with a refreshing and energizing morning boost smoothie. This invigorating concoction will not only give you a vibrant start to your day but also provide essential nutrients.

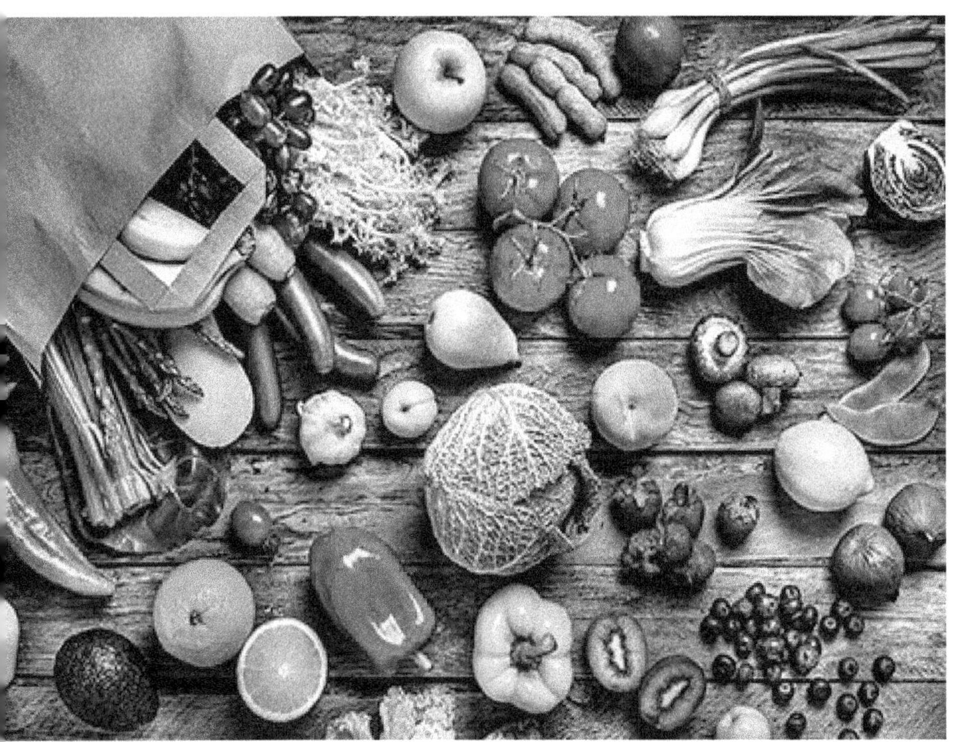

Ingredients:

cups of fresh baby spinach

ripe banana

tablespoon of pineapple chunks

tablespoon of chia seeds

cup of coconut water

Instructions:

GREEN SMOOTHIE REVOLUTION

Thoroughly wash the baby spinach, ensuring the remo
of any tough stems.

Peel the banana and add in a blender, combine the ba
spinach, banana, pineapple chunks, chia seeds, and
coconut water.

Blend until smooth and creamy.

Pour the smoothie into a glass and savor the refreshin
green goodness.

Benefits: This morning boost smoothie is packed with
important nutrients such as vitamins, minerals, and
antioxidants. The banana and pineapple provide natura
sweetness and an extra dose of vitamin C. Baby spinac
contributes iron and fiber for a healthy boost. Chia see
offer omega-3 fatty acids and additional fiber to sustai
energy levels throughout the day.

For Day 2, focus on detoxifying and cleansing your boc
with a green smoothie. This recipe supports your body
natural detoxification processes and promotes a health
digestive system.

redients:

ups of kale leaves

ucumber

reen apple

ce of 1/2 lemon

nch piece of ginger

up of coconut water

tructions:

move the fibrous stems from the kale leaves and wash

m thoroughly.

d the cucumber and green apple

el and grate the ginger.

a blender, combine all and add water.

nd until smooth and well combined.

ur the smoothie into a glass and enjoy the revitalizing

/or.

nefits: This green cleanse smoothie is rich in

chlorophyll and antioxidants. Kale supports liver detoxification, while cucumber helps hydrate the body and flush out toxins. Green apple adds fiber and vitamin C. Ginger and lemon juice aid digestion and boost metabolism.

For Day 3, strengthen your immune system with a vibrant and nutrient-packed smoothie. This delicious blend provides a boost to your overall health and enhances your body's natural defenses.

Ingredients:

2 cups of chopped baby spinach

1 ripe mango, peeled and sliced

1 small orange, peeled and segmented

1/2 cup of Greek yogurt

1 teaspoon of honey

1/2 cup of almond milk

Instructions:

an the baby spinach thoroughly and remove any

ms.

e the peeled mango.

el the orange

a blender, combine the baby spinach, mango, orange

gments, Greek yogurt, honey, and almond milk.

end until smooth and creamy.

ur the smoothie into a glass and indulge in the

mune-boosting goodness.

nefits: This smoothie is packed with vitamins,

nerals, and antioxidants to support your immune

stem. Baby spinach provides vitamin C, while mango

d orange contribute additional vitamin C and other

mune-boosting nutrients. Greek yogurt offers

obiotics for a healthy gut, and honey adds antibacterial

d antiviral properties.

Smoothie for Radiant Skin on Day 6

Indulge in a skin-nourishing smoothie that will hydrate a
enhance your complexion. This recipe is brimming w
ingredients that promote a radiant and healthy appearar
for your skin.

Ingredients:

2 cups of fresh spinach, chopped

1/2 ounce of fresh strawberries

1/2 cup of fresh blueberries

1/4 cup of plain Greek yogurt

1 teaspoon of flaxseed oil

1 cup of coconut water

Instructions:

Thoroughly wash the spinach and remove any tou
stems.

se the strawberries and blueberries.

nbine the spinach, strawberries, blueberries, Greek
gurt, flaxseed oil, and coconut water in a blender.

nd until smooth and well combined.

ur the smoothie into a glass and relish in its skin-
urishing benefits.

nefits: This smoothie is packed with antioxidants and
crients that are beneficial for your skin. Spinach is rich
vitamins A and C, essential for maintaining healthy skin
d collagen production. Strawberries and blueberries are
ded with antioxidants that protect cells from free radical
mage and slow down the aging process. Greek yogurt
ovides probiotics for a healthy gut-skin connection.
xseed oil, abundant in omega-3 fatty acids, promotes
n hydration and suppleness.

noothie for Muscle Recovery on Day 7

Accelerate your muscle recovery process with a nutritio
smoothie designed to support and repair your muscl
This recipe incorporates vital nutrients that aid in mus
reconstruction and rejuvenation.

Ingredients:

2 cups of kale leaves

1 ripe banana

1/2 cup of plain Greek yogurt

1 tablespoon of almond butter

1/2 teaspoon of honey

1/2 cup of almond milk

Instructions:

Wash the kale leaves thoroughly and remove the tou
stems. Peel and chop the banana.

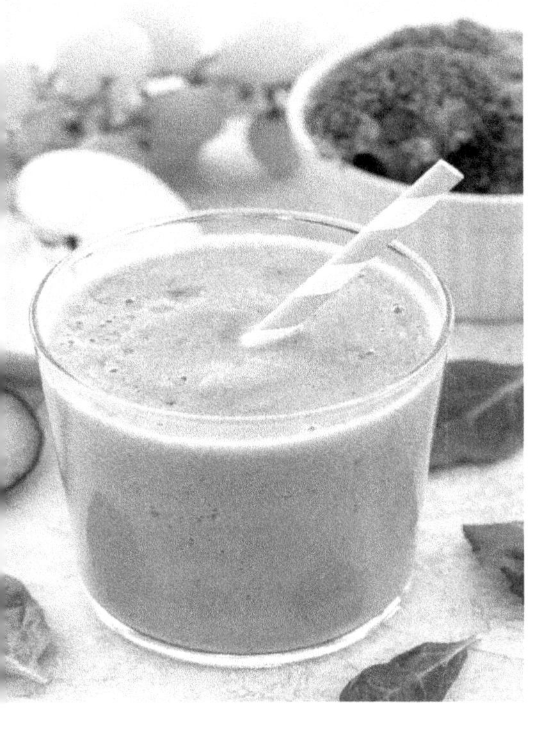

Blend the kale leaves, banana, Greek yogurt, almond butter, honey, and almond milk until smooth. Serve immediately.

Benefits: This muscle recovery smoothie is packed with nutrients that assist in muscle repair and healing. Kale contains antioxidants and anti-inflammatory compounds that reduce exercise-induced inflammation.

Bananas provide potassium, an electrolyte crucial for proper muscle function. Greek yogurt is a rich source of protein, essential for muscle tissue regeneration. Almond butter offers healthy fats and additional protein, while honey replenishes energy stores.

Smoothie for Mental Clarity on Day 8

Boost your cognitive function and improve mental cla
with a refreshing smoothie that nourishes your brain. T
recipe provides essential nutrients for optimal brain hea
and enhanced focus.

Ingredients:

2 cups of baby spinach

1/2 cup of blueberries

1/2 ripe avocado

1 teaspoon of coconut oil

1 teaspoon of chia seeds

1 cup of coconut water

Instructions:

oroughly wash the baby spinach and remove any tough
:ms.

ise the blueberries.

t the avocado in half, remove the pit, and scoop out the
sh.

 a blender, combine the baby spinach, blueberries,
ocado, chia seeds, and coconut water. Blend until
iooth.

ur the smoothie into a glass and enjoy the brain-
osting benefits.

nefits: This smoothie is loaded with components that
omote brain health and cognitive function. Baby spinach
rich in essential vitamins and minerals, including folate,
cessary for neurotransmitter function. Blueberries are
cked with antioxidants that protect brain cells from
idative stress.

ocado provides beneficial fats, such as omega-3 fatty
ids, crucial for optimal brain function. Coconut oil

contains medium-chain triglycerides (MCTs), known
enhance mental clarity and focus. Chia seeds contrib
omega-3 fatty acids and fiber, providing sustained ener

Smoothie for Heart Health on Day 9

Take care of your heart and maintain cardiovascular hea
with a nutrient-rich smoothie designed to support
healthy heart. This recipe provides the necessary nutrie
to keep your heart strong and vibrant.

Ingredients:

2 cups of fresh spinach

1/2 cup of frozen berries (blueberries, strawberries,
raspberries)

1/2 ripe banana

1 teaspoon of ground flaxseed

1 tablespoon of raw cacao powder

1 cup of almond milk

tructions:

oroughly wash the spinach and remove any tough
ms.

using fresh berries, rinse them; if using frozen berries,
rost them.

el and chop the banana.

mbine the spinach, berries, banana, ground flaxseed,
v cacao powder, and almond milk in a blender. Blend
til smooth.

ur the smoothie into a glass and savor its deliciousness
it supports your heart.

nefits: This smoothie is packed with ingredients that
omote cardiovascular fitness and heart health. Spinach,
h its antioxidants and minerals like potassium, helps
luce blood pressure. Berries contain anthocyanins,
tent antioxidants that reduce inflammation and improve

blood vessel function. Bananas contribute natu
sweetness and potassium, while ground flaxseed off
omega-3 fatty acids and fiber. Raw cacao powder provid
flavonoids that benefit heart health.

Smoothie for a Restful Sleep on Day 10

Unwind and prepare for a peaceful night's sleep with
calming and sleep-inducing smoothie. This rec
incorporates ingredients known for their relax
properties to promote a refreshing and restful sleep.

Ingredients:

2 cups of tart cherry juice

1 small ripe banana

1/2 cup of plain Greek yogurt

1 tablespoon of almond butter

1 teaspoon of honey (optional)

1/2 teaspoon of cinnamon powder

tructions:

a blender, combine the tart cherry juice, banana, Greek
urt, almond butter, honey (if desired), and cinnamon
vder. Blend until smooth.

ur the smoothie into a glass and enjoy its sedative
perties.

efits: This tranquil sleep smoothie contains
nponents that help you de-stress and improve the
ality of your sleep. Tart cherry juice is a natural source
melatonin, a hormone that regulates sleep-wake cycles.
nanas provide potassium and magnesium, minerals that
m the nerves and relax muscles.

ek yogurt contains calcium, essential for melatonin
duction. Almond butter supplies beneficial fats and
tein to sustain energy levels during sleep. Cinnamon
only adds flavor but also helps regulate blood sugar
els, reducing sleep disturbances.

GREEN SMOOTHIE REVOLUTION

Congratulations on completing the 10-day green smoothie transformation! By incorporating these nutritious and health-promoting smoothies into your daily routine, you've taken a significant step towards reshaping your body and adopting a healthier lifestyle.

Remember, these smoothie recipes are meant to complement a well-rounded diet and healthy lifestyle.

3.3 Tracking Your Progress

It's essential to keep a close eye on your progress as you embark on your green smoothie revolution. This will help you stay motivated and witness the positive changes happening within your body. Monitoring your progress allows you to evaluate your advancements and make any necessary adjustments along the way. Here are some practical methods to track your journey:

Journaling: Throughout the 10-day transformation, maintain a journal where you can record your daily experiences, observations, and emotions. Note any provements in your mood, digestion, energy levels, anges in your physique, or any other relevant servations. This journal will serve as a valuable erence point, allowing you to reflect on how far you've ne.

asurements and Weigh-ins: Before starting the gram, consider taking measurements and weighing urself to track your progress towards your weight loss body transformation goals. Measure key areas such as ur waist, hips, chest, and arms.

cord your starting weight and monitor changes by ighing yourself every few days or at regular intervals. member that progress goes beyond the numbers on the ale; it also includes how you feel and how well your thes fit.

gress Photos: Visual evidence can be a powerful tool to asure your physical transformation. Take "before" otos from various angles on Day 1 and repeat the cess on Day 10. By comparing the before and after ages side by side, you can clearly see any changes in

your body shape, skin tone, or overall appearance. The
visual reminders can be highly motivating and inspiring.

Assessing Energy and Well-being: Regularly evaluate yo
energy levels, mood, sleep quality, and overall well-be
throughout the 10-day journey. Rate them on a scale o
to 10 and make notes of any changes or improveme
you observe.

This self-assessment will give you a better understandi
of how consuming green smoothies positively impacts yo
vitality and quality of life.

Feedback from Others: Pay attention to comments a
suggestions from those around you, such as friends a
coworkers. They may notice changes in your appearan
energy levels, or mood. Their insights can provide valua
additional perspective on the positive transformatio
taking place within you.

Celebrate Achievements and Milestones: Celebrate yo
past accomplishments and significant milestones as y
progress. Recognize and reward yourself for completi
the full 10-day challenge, achieving weight loss targe

eriencing increased energy levels, or overcoming sonal challenges. Treat yourself to non-food-related ards that align with your goals and bring you joy.

member that monitoring your progress isn't just about ching a specific destination; it's also about appreciating journey that got you there. Every step forward resents a victory and an opportunity for personal wth.

tracking your progress, making necessary adjustments, ying motivated, and celebrating positive improvements, can continue to thrive in your commitment to the en smoothie revolution.

ep up the excellent work, and here's to a happier, althier you!

Beyond the 10-Day Challenge: Explorir

Chapter 4

Congratulations on successfully completing the 10-da
green smoothie revolution! By now, you've likely
experienced the numerous benefits of incorporating
green smoothies into your routine. In this chapter, we
will delve into how you can continue enjoying these
benefits beyond the initial challenge, making green
smoothies a permanent and enjoyable part of your
lifestyle.

4.1 Embracing the Benefits of Green Smoothies for Your Daily Life

After completing the 10-day challenge, you might be
wondering how to continue reaping the rewards of gre
smoothies. Here are some suggestions to help you
effortlessly integrate healthy green smoothies into you

ryday routine:

ablish a habit: consistency is key. Set a specific time
h day for your green smoothie, whether it's part of
ır breakfast routine, a mid-morning snack, or a post-
kout replenishment. Establishing a ritual will help you
y committed to your green smoothie journey.

n and Prepare: To simplify your adherence to a green
oothie regimen, it's helpful to plan your smoothie
ipes in advance. Create a weekly meal plan, make a
pping list, and ensure you have all the necessary
redients on hand.

ısider prepping components in advance, such as
shing and slicing greens and chopping fruits, and
ring them in convenient containers for quick and easy
nding.

eriment with Ingredients: Keep the experience of
king green smoothies fun and exciting by exploring

different flavors and variations. Try various combinatic
of fruits, veggies, and superfoods to discover your
favorite blends. Don't hesitate to be creative and use
seasonal produce or unique ingredients to keep your
taste buds engaged and intrigued.

Enhance Nutritional Content: While green smoothies a
already packed with healthy ingredients, you can furth
boost their nutritional value. Consider adding plant-ba
protein powders like pea or hemp protein to increase
your protein intake.

Incorporating a tablespoon of flaxseeds or chia seeds
enhance fiber and omega-3 fatty acids. For additional
nutritional benefits, explore superfoods such as spirulir
wheatgrass, or maca powder.

4.2 Exploring Different Tastes and Variation

Now that you have a basic understanding of green
smoothies, it's time to broaden your horizons and
venture into various taste combinations and variations

h the sample given below:

opical Paradise Smoothie: Blend spinach, mango,
neapple, a splash of coconut water, and a squeeze of
ne for a delightful tropical twist.

eamy Green Avocado Smoothie: Create a rich and
tisfying treat by blending kale, avocado, banana,
mond milk, and a tablespoon of almond butter for
eamy, green goodness.

rry-Licious Spinach Smoothie: Blend spinach, a variety
berries (strawberries, blueberries, and raspberries),
eek yogurt, and a drizzle of honey for a vibrant,
tioxidant-rich treat.

een Detox Smoothie: Detoxify your body and boost
erall health by blending spinach, cucumber, celery,
mon juice, ginger, and coconut water until smooth.

4.3 Green Vegetable Smoothies for Special Dietary Needs

Green smoothies are versatile enough to cater to vario dietary requirements and personal tastes. Here are sor ideas for specific dietary considerations:

Vegan/Vegetarian Options: Replace dairy milk with pla based alternatives such as oat milk, almond milk, or coconut milk. Substitute Greek yogurt with dairy-free options like coconut yogurt or soy yogurt.

Gluten-Free Alternatives: Stick to gluten-free ingredien like spinach, kale, fruits, and uncontaminated oats. Avc barley grass and wheatgrass powders if you are gluten sensitive.

Nut-Free Options: Instead of nut milk and nut butter, t oat milk, rice milk, or seed butter (sunflower seed, pumpkin seed). Incorporate nutrient-rich seeds like chi seeds or hemp seeds for added texture and nutrients.

v-Sugar Choices: opt for low-sugar fruits like berries, en apples, or citrus fruits as the foundation of your oothies. Avoid adding extra sweeteners and rely on natural sweetness of the fruits.

member, even after completing the 10-day challenge, en smoothies can continue to nourish your body and hance your overall well-being.

nsistently incorporating them into your routine, perimenting with different flavors, and customizing m to fit your dietary needs will help you reap long-term nefits. Embrace the flexibility and limitless possibilities green smoothies as you embark on a lifelong journey vards optimal health and energy.

re's to a thriving future filled with green goodness!

Conclusion

In conclusion, the 10-day green smoothie transformat
has provided you with a diverse range of smoothie recip
that offer numerous health benefits. By incorporat
these nutrient-rich concoctions into your daily routine, y
have taken a proactive step towards improving yo
overall well-being.

Throughout the 10 days, you have explored smoothies t
cater to specific areas of health, including radiant sk
muscle recovery, mental clarity, heart health, and rest
sleep. Each smoothie recipe has been carefully crafted
include ingredients that target the respective aspect
health, providing you with a delicious and convenient w
to nourish your body.

smoothies for radiant skin have supplied your skin
antioxidants, vitamins, and probiotics, promoting a
complexion and combating signs of aging. The
recovery smoothies have aided in the repair and
rejuvenation of your muscles, supporting your fitness
journey.

smoothies for mental clarity have given your brain the
essential nutrients it needs for optimal cognitive function
and focus. The heart-healthy smoothies have contributed
cardiovascular fitness and the maintenance of a strong
heart.

Lastly, the sleep-inducing smoothies have helped you
wind and enjoy restful nights of sleep, promoting overall
relaxation and well-being.

It's important to remember that these smoothie recipes
should be part of a well-rounded diet and a healthy
lifestyle.

GREEN SMOOTHIE REVOLUTION

While they offer numerous health benefits, it is alwa
advisable to consult with a qualified medical practitior
before making significant changes to your diet, especia
if you have any preexisting health concerns or speci
dietary requirements.

By completing this 10-day green smoothie transformatic
you have shown dedication to your health and have tak
a significant step towards adopting a healthier way of li

Enjoy the continued benefits of these nutritious a
delicious smoothies as you prioritize your well-being a
continue on your journey to a healthier you.

Cheers to your success and a vibrant, health-conscio
future!

www.ingramcontent.com/pod-product-compliance
Lightning Source LLC
Chambersburg PA
CBHW072342270726

48659CB00023B/2198